Mediterranean Dash Diet Recipe Book

Don't Miss These Tasty and Affordable Recipes to Make Incredible Mediterranean Dash Diet Meals

Kathyrn Solano

© Copyright 2021 - All rights reserved.

The content contained within this book may not be reproduced, duplicated or transmitted without direct written permission from the author or the publisher.

Under no circumstances will any blame or legal responsibility be held against the publisher, or author, for any damages, reparation, or monetary loss due to the information contained within this book. Either directly or indirectly.

Legal Notice:

This book is copyright protected. This book is only for personal use. You cannot amend, distribute, sell, use, quote or paraphrase any part, or the content within this book, without the consent of the author or publisher.

Disclaimer Notice:

Please note the information contained within this document is for educational and entertainment purposes only. All effort has been executed to present accurate, up to date, and reliable, complete information. No warranties of any kind are declared or implied. Readers acknowledge that the author is not engaging in the rendering of legal, financial, medical or professional advice. The content within this book has been derived from various sources.

Please consult a licensed professional before attempting any techniques outlined in this book.

By reading this document, the reader agrees that under no circumstances is the author responsible for any losses, direct or indirect, which are incurred as a result of the use of information contained within this document, including, but not limited to, — errors, omissions, or inaccuracies.

Table of contents

BREAKFAST & LUNCH 6
    PEARL COUSCOUS SALAD 6
    RUM-RAISIN ARBORIO PUDDING 8
    BREAKFAST CAULIFLOWER RICE BOWL 10
    SAVORY CUCUMBER-DILL YOGURT 11
    CRANBERRY SPICE TEA 13
    HEALTHY DRY FRUIT PORRIDGE 14
    PESTO SCRAMBLED EGGS 15
    BREAKFAST JALAPENO EGG CUPS 16
    QUINOA BAKE WITH BANANA 18
    PEAR AND MANGO SMOOTHIE 20
    CAPPUCCINO MUFFINS 21
    FETA SPINACH EGG CUPS 23
    CHOCOLATE ALMOND BUTTER DIP 24
    SUN DRIED TOMATOES, DILL AND FETA OMELETTE CASSEROLE 25

LUNCH AND DINNER RECIPES 27
    BEEF SAUSAGE PANCAKES 27
    CHICKEN SAUSAGE, ARTICHOKE, KALE, AND WHITE BEAN GRATIN 29
    STEAK AND VEGGIES 31
    LENTIL AND ROASTED CARROT SALAD WITH HERBS AND FETA 33
    CINNAMON SQUASH SOUP 35
    CREAMY CHICKEN 38
    CHICKEN DRUMMIES WITH PEACH GLAZE 39
    BERRY COMPOTE WITH ORANGE MINT INFUSION 41
    QUINOA BRUSCHETTA SALAD 43
    ZESTY LEMON PARMESAN CHICKEN AND ZUCCHINI NOODLES 45
    THREE CITRUS SAUCE SCALLOPS 46
    STEAMED MUSSELS TOPPED WITH WINE SAUCE 49
    SPICE POTATO SOUP 51
    SPICY CAJUN SHRIMP 53
    PAN-SEARED SALMON 55
    PASTA FAGGIOLI SOUP 56
    FATTOUSH SALAD 58
    ROAST CHICKEN 60
    CHICKEN EGGPLANT 62
    GRILLED STEAK 64
    BEEF AND VEGGIE LASAGNA 65
    GREEK SHRIMP AND FARRO BOWLS 68

ASPARAGUS SALMON FILLETS 70
GRILLED CALAMARI WITH BERRIES 71
ITALIAN SAUSAGE AND VEGGIE PIZZA PASTA 73
BAKED CHICKEN THIGHS WITH LEMON, OLIVES, AND BRUSSELS SPROUTS 76
SLOW COOKER LAMB, HERB, AND BEAN STEW 78
HOLIDAY CHICKEN SALAD 80
COSTA BRAVA CHICKEN 81
ONE SKILLET GREEK LEMON CHICKEN AND RICE 83
TROUT WITH WILTED GREENS 86
ONE SKILLET CHICKEN IN ROASTED RED PEPPER SAUCE 88
MEDITERRANEAN MINESTRONE SOUP 90
BAKED SHRIMP STEW 92
MEDITERRANEAN PORK PITA SANDWICH 94

SAUCES AND DRESSINGS RECIPES 96

POMEGRANATE VINAIGRETTE 96
GREEN OLIVE AND SPINACH TAPENADE 98

GREAT MEDITERRANEAN DIET RECIPES 99

GRILLED LEMON CHICKEN SKEWERS 99
BLACK-EYED PEAS SALAD 101
CHICKEN SHAWARMA PITAS 103
SAUTÉED CHICKEN WITH OLIVES CAPERS AND LEMONS 105
SPANISH RICE CASSEROLE WITH CHEESY BEEF 107

BREAKFAST & LUNCH

Pearl Couscous Salad

Servings: 6
Cooking Time: 10 Minutes

Ingredients:

lemon juice, 1 large lemon

1/3 cup extra-virgin olive oil

1 teaspoon dill weed

1 teaspoon garlic powder

salt

pepper

2 cups Pearl Couscous

2 tablespoons extra virgin olive oil

2 cups grape tomatoes, halved

water as needed

1/3 cup red onions, finely chopped

½ English cucumber, finely chopped

1 15-ounce can chickpeas

1 14-ounce can artichoke hearts, roughly chopped

½ cup pitted Kalamata olives

15-20 pieces fresh basil leaves, roughly torn and chopped

3 ounces fresh mozzarella

Directions:

Start by preparing the vinaigrette by mixing all Ingredients: in a bowl. Set aside.

Heat olive oil in a medium-sized heavy pot over medium heat.

Add couscous and cook until golden brown.

Add 3 cups of boiling water and cook the couscous according to package instructions.

Once done, drain in a colander and put it to the side.

In a large mixing bowl, add the rest of the Ingredients: except the cheese and basil.

Add the cooked couscous, basil, and mix everything well.

Give the vinaigrette a gentle stir and whisk it into the couscous salad. Mix well.

Adjust/add seasoning as desired.

Add mozzarella cheese.

Garnish with some basil.

Enjoy!

Nutrition Info: Calories: 578, Total Fat: 25.3g, Saturated Fat: 4.6, Cholesterol: 8 mg, Sodium: 268 mg, Total Carbohydrate: 70.1g, Dietary Fiber: 17.5 g, Total Sugars: 10.8 g, Protein: 23.4 g, Vitamin D: 0 mcg, Calcium: 150 mg, Iron: 6 mg, Potassium: 1093 mg

Rum-raisin Arborio Pudding

Servings: 2

Cooking Time: 4 Hours

Ingredients:

¾ cup Arborio rice

1 can evaporated milk

½ cup raisins

¼ teaspoon nutmeg, grated

1½ cups water

1/3 cup sugar

¼ cup dark rum

sea salt or plain salt

Directions:

Start by mixing rum and raisins in a bowl and set aside.

Then, heat the evaporated milk and water in a saucepan and then simmer.

Now, add sugar and stir until dissolved.

Finally, convert this milk mixture into a slow cooker and stir in rice and salt.

Cook on low heat for hours.

Now, stir in the raisin mixture and nutmeg and let sit for 10 minutes.

Serve warm.

Nutrition Info: Calories: 3, Total Fat: 10.1g, Saturated Fat: 5.9, Cholesterol: 36 mg, Sodium: 161 mg, Total Carbohydrate: 131.5 g, Dietary Fiber: 3.3 g, Total Sugars: 54.8 g, Protein: 14.4 g, Vitamin D: 0 mcg, Calcium: 372 mg, Iron: 2 mg, Potassium: 7

Breakfast Cauliflower Rice Bowl

Servings: 6

Cooking Time: 12 Minutes

Ingredients:

1 cup cauliflower rice

1/2 tsp red pepper flakes

1 1/2 tsp curry powder

1/2 tbsp ginger, grated

1 cup vegetable stock

4 tomatoes, chopped

3 cups broccoli, chopped

Pepper

Salt

Directions: Spray instant pot from inside with cooking spray. Add all ingredients into the instant pot and stir well. Seal pot with lid and cook on high for 12 minutes. Once done, allow to release pressure naturally for 10 minutes then release remaining using quick release. Remove lid. Stir and serve.

Nutrition Info: Calories: 44;Fat: 0.8 g; Carbohydrates: 8.2 g; Sugar: 3.8 g; Protein: 2.8 g; Cholesterol: 0 mg

Savory Cucumber-dill Yogurt

Servings: 4

Cooking Time: 10 Minutes

Ingredients:

2 cups low-fat (2%) plain Greek yogurt

4 teaspoons minced shallot

4 teaspoons freshly squeezed lemon juice

¼ cup chopped fresh dill

2 teaspoons olive oil

¼ teaspoon kosher salt

Pinch freshly ground black pepper

2 cups chopped Persian cucumbers (about 4 medium cucumbers)

Directions:

Combine the yogurt, shallot, lemon juice, dill, oil, salt, and pepper in a large bowl.

Taste the mixture and add another pinch of salt if needed.

Scoop ½ cup of yogurt into each of 4 containers.

Place ½ cup of chopped cucumbers in each of 4 separate small containers or resealable sandwich bags.

STORAGE: Store covered containers in the refrigerator for up to 5 days.

Nutrition Info: Total calories: 127; Total fat: 5g; Saturated fat: 2g; Sodium: 200mg; Carbohydrates: 9g; Fiber: 2g; Protein: 11g

Cranberry Spice Tea

Servings: 2

Cooking Time: 18 Minutes

Ingredients:

1-ounce cranberries

½ lemon, juice, and zest

1 cinnamon stick

2 teabags

½ inch ginger, peeled and grated

raw honey to taste

3 cups water

Directions:

Start by adding all the Ingredients: except honey into a pot or saucepan. Bring to a boil and then simmer for about 115 minutes. Strain and serve the tea. Add honey or any other sweetener of your preference. Enjoy.

Nutrition Info: Calories: 38, Total Fat: 0.3g, Saturated Fat: 0.1, Cholesterol: 0 mg, Sodium: 2 mg, Total Carbohydrate: 10 g, Dietary Fiber: 4.9 g, Total Sugars: 1.1 g, Protein: 0.7 g, Vitamin D: 0 mcg, Calcium: 77 mg, Iron: 1 mg, Potassium: 110 mg

Healthy Dry Fruit Porridge

Servings: 6

Cooking Time: 8 Hours

Ingredients:

2 cups steel-cut oats

1/8 tsp ground nutmeg

1 tsp vanilla

1 1/2 tsp cinnamon

1/2 cup dry apricots, chopped

1/2 cup dry cranberries, chopped

1/2 cup dates, chopped

1/2 cup raisins

8 cups of water

Pinch of salt

Directions: Spray instant pot from inside with cooking spray. Add all ingredients into the instant pot and stir well. Seal the pot with a lid and select slow cook mode and cook on low for 8 hours. Stir well and serve.

Nutrition Info: Calories: 196;Fat: 2 g; Carbohydrates: 42 g; Sugar: 18.4 g; Protein: 4.g;Cholesterol: 0 mg

Pesto Scrambled Eggs

Servings: 2

Cooking Time: 10 Minutes

Ingredients:

5 eggs

2 tablespoons butter

2 tablespoons pesto

4 tablespoons milk

salt to taste

pepper to taste

Directions:

Beat the eggs into a bowl and add salt and pepper as per your taste. Then, heat a pan and add the butter, then the eggs, stirring continuously. While stirring continuously, add the pesto. Switch off the heat and quickly add the creamed milk and mix it well with eggs. Serve hot.

Nutrition Info: Calories: 342, Total Fat: 29.8g, Saturated Fat: 12.3, Cholesterol: 44mg, Sodium: 345 mg, Total Carbohydrate: 3.4g, Dietary Fiber: 0.3 g, Total Sugars: 3.2 g, Protein: 16.8 g, Vitamin D: 47 mcg, Calcium: 148 mg, Iron: 2 mg, Potassium: 168 mg

Breakfast Jalapeno Egg Cups

Servings: 6

Cooking Time: 8 Minutes

Ingredients:

12 eggs, lightly beaten

1/4 tsp garlic powder

1/2 tsp lemon pepper seasoning

3 jalapeno peppers, chopped

1 cup cheddar cheese, shredded

Pepper

Salt

Directions:

Pour 1/2 cups of water into the instant pot then place steamer rack in the pot.

In a bowl, whisk eggs with lemon pepper seasoning, garlic powder, pepper, and salt.

Stir in jalapenos and cheese.

Pour mixture between six jars and seal jar with a lid.

Place jars on top of the rack in the instant pot.

Seal pot with a lid and select manual and set timer for 8 minutes.

Once done, allow to release pressure naturally for 10 minutes then release remaining using quick release. Remove lid.

Serve and enjoy.

Nutrition Info: Calories: 212;Fat: 15.2 g; Carbohydrates: 3.2 g; Sugar: 2.1 g; Protein: 16.1 g; Cholesterol: 347 mg

Quinoa Bake With Banana

Servings: 8

Cooking Time: 1 Hour 20 Minutes

Ingredients:

3 cups medium over-ripe Bananas, mashed

1/4 cup molasses

1/4 cup pure maple syrup

1 tbsp cinnamon

2 tsp raw vanilla extract

1 tsp ground ginger

1 tsp ground cloves

1/2 tsp ground allspice

1/2 tsp salt

1 cup quinoa, uncooked

2 1/2 cups unsweetened vanilla almond milk

1/4 cup slivered almonds

Directions:

In the bottom of a 2 2-3-quart casserole dish, mix together the mashed banana, maple syrup, cinnamon, vanilla extract, ginger, cloves, allspice, molasses, and salt until well mixed

Add in the quinoa, stir until the quinoa is evenly in the banana mixture.

Whisk in the almond milk, mix until well combined, cover and refrigerate overnight or bake immediately

Heat oven to 350 degrees F

Whisk the quinoa mixture making sure it doesn't settle to the bottom

Cover the pan with tinfoil and bake until the liquid is absorbed, and the top of the quinoa is set, about 1 hour to 1 hour and 15 mins

Turn the oven to high broil, uncover the pan, sprinkle with sliced almonds, and lightly press them into the quinoa

Broil until the almonds just turn golden brown, about 2-4 minutes, watching closely, as they burn quickly

Allow to cool for 10 minutes then slice the quinoa bake

Distribute the quinoa bake among the containers, store in the fridge for 3-4 days

Nutrition Info: Calories:213;Carbs: 41g;Total Fat: 4g;Protein: 5g

Pear And Mango Smoothie

Servings: 1

Cooking Time: 10 Minutes

Ingredients:

½ peeled, pitted, and chopped mango

2 cubes of ice

1 ripe, cored, and chopped pear

½ cup of plain Greek yogurt

1 cup chopped kale

Directions:

In a blender, combine the mango, ice cubes, pear, yogurt, and kale.

Blend until the mixture is smooth and thick.

Serve and enjoy!

Nutrition Info: calories: 293, fats: 8 grams, carbohydrates: 53 grams, protein: 8 grams.

Cappuccino Muffins

Servings: 2

Cooking Time: 20 Minutes

Ingredients:

2 1/3 cups all-purpose flour

2 tsp baking powder

1 tsp salt

1 tsp ground cinnamon

¾ cup hot water

2 tbsp espresso powder or instant coffee

2 eggs

1 cup sugar

¾ cup vegetable oil

1/3 cup mini chocolate chips

¼ cup milk

Directions:

Preheat oven to 425 degree F

In a medium bowl, whisk together the flour, baking powder, salt and cinnamon, set aside

In a small bowl, combine the hot water and espresso powder, stir to dissolve, add milk, stir to combine and set aside

In a large bowl, whisk together eggs, sugar and oil, slowly add the coffee mixture, and stir to combine Then add in the dry ingredients in thirds, whisking gently until smooth

Add in the chocolate chips, stir to combine

Place the muffin papers in a 12-cup muffin tin

Fill each cup half way

Bake for 17-20 minutes, until risen and set

Allow to cool completely before slicing

Wrap the slices in plastic wrap and then aluminum foil and store in fridge for up to 4-5 days

To Serve: Remove the aluminum foil and plastic wrap, and microwave for 2 minutes, then allow to rest for 30 seconds, enjoy!

Nutrition Info: (1 muffin): Calories:201;Carbs: 29g;Total Fat: 8g;Protein: 2g

Feta Spinach Egg Cups

Servings: 4

Cooking Time: 8 Minutes

Ingredients:

6 eggs

1/4 tsp garlic powder

1 tomato, chopped

1/4 cup feta cheese, crumbled

1 cup spinach, chopped

1/2 cup mozzarella cheese, shredded

Salt; pepper to taste

Directions:

Pour 1/2 cups of water into the instant pot then place steamer rack in the pot. In a bowl, whisk eggs with garlic powder, pepper, and salt. Add remaining ingredients and stir well.

Spray four ramekins with cooking spray. Pour egg mixture into the ramekins and place ramekins on top of the rack. Seal pot with lid and cook on high for 8 minutes. Once done, release pressure using quick release. Remove lid. Serve and enjoy.

Nutrition Info: Calories: 134;Fat: 3 g; Carbohydrates: 2 g; Sugar: 1.4 g; Protein: 11 g; Cholesterol: 256 mg

Chocolate Almond Butter Dip

Servings: 5

Cooking Time: 10 Minutes

Ingredients:

1 cup of Plain Greek Yogurt

½ cup almond butter

1/3 cup chocolate hazelnut spread

1 tablespoon honey

1 teaspoon vanilla

sliced up fruits as you desire, such as pears, apples, apricots, bananas, etc.

Directions:

Take a medium-sized bowl and add all Ingredients: except the fruit. Take an immersion blender and blend everything well until a smooth dip forms. Alternatively, you can Directions: the Ingredients: in a food processor as well. Serve with your favorite fruit slices!

Nutrition Info: Calories: 148, Total Fat: 7.3 g, Saturated Fat: 1.8 g, Cholesterol: 1 mg, Sodium: 26 mg, Total Carbohydrate: 17 g, Dietary Fiber: 0.7 g, Total Sugars: 15 g, Protein: 5.9 g, Vitamin D: 0 mcg, Calcium: 37 mg, Iron: 0 mg, Potassium: 15 mg

Sun Dried Tomatoes, Dill And Feta Omelette Casserole

Servings: 6

Cooking Time: 40

Ingredients:

12 large eggs

2 cups whole milk

8 oz fresh spinach

2 cloves garlic, minced

12 oz artichoke salad with olives and peppers, drained and chopped

5 oz sun dried tomato feta cheese, crumbled

1 tbsp fresh chopped dill or 1 tsp dried dill

1 tsp dried oregano

1 tsp lemon pepper

1 tsp salt

4 tsp olive oil, divided

Directions:

Preheat oven to 375 degrees F

Chop the fresh herbs and artichoke salad

In a skillet over medium heat, add 1 tbsp olive oil

Sauté the spinach and garlic until wilted, about 3 minutes

Oil a 9x13 inch baking dish, layer the spinach and artichoke salad evenly in the dish

In a medium bowl, whisk together the eggs, milk, herbs, salt and lemon pepper

Pour the egg mixture over vegetables, sprinkle with feta cheese

Bake in the center of the oven for 35-40 minutes until firm in the center

Allow to cool, slice a and distribute among the storage containers. Store for 2-3 days or freeze for 3 months

To Serve: Reheat in the microwave for 30 seconds or until heated through or in the toaster oven for 5 minutes or until heated through

Nutrition Info: Calories:196;Total Carbohydrates: 5g;Total Fat: 2g;Protein: 10g

LUNCH AND DINNER RECIPES

Beef Sausage Pancakes

Servings: 2

Cooking Time: 30 Minutes

Ingredients:

4 gluten-free Italian beef sausages, sliced

1 tablespoon olive oil

1/3 large red bell peppers, seeded and sliced thinly

1/3 cup spinach

¾ teaspoon garlic powder

1/3 large green bell peppers, seeded and sliced thinly

¾ cup heavy whipped cream

Salt and black pepper, to taste

Directions:

Mix together all the ingredients in a bowl except whipped cream and keep aside.

Put butter and half of the mixture in a skillet and cook for about 6 minutes on both sides.

Repeat with the remaining mixture and dish out.

Beat whipped cream in another bowl until smooth.

Serve the beef sausage pancakes with whipped cream.

For meal prepping, it is compulsory to gently slice the sausages before mixing with other ingredients.

Nutrition Info: Calories: 415 ;Carbohydrates: ;Protein: 29.5g;Fat: 31.6g ;Sugar: 4.3g;Sodium: 1040mg

Chicken Sausage, Artichoke, Kale, And White Bean Gratin

Servings: 8

Cooking Time: 45 Minutes

Ingredients:

2 teaspoons olive oil, plus 2 tablespoons

1 small yellow onion, chopped (about 2 cups)

1 (12-ounce) package fully cooked chicken-apple sausage, sliced

1 bunch kale, stemmed and chopped (6 to 7 cups)

½ cup dry white wine, such as sauvignon blanc

4 ounces soft goat cheese

2 (15.5-ounce) cans cannellini or great northern beans, drained and rinsed

1 (14-ounce) can quartered artichoke hearts

1 (14.5-ounce) can no-salt-added diced tomatoes

1 teaspoon herbes de Provence

¼ teaspoon kosher salt

1 cup panko bread crumbs

1 teaspoon garlic powder

Directions:

Preheat the oven to 350°F. Lightly oil a -by-9-inch glass or ceramic baking dish.

Heat teaspoons of oil in a 12-inch skillet over medium-high heat. When the oil is shimmering, add the onion and cook for 2 minutes. Add the sausage and brown for 3 minutes. Add the kale and cook until wilted, about 3 more minutes. Add the wine and cook for 1 additional minute.

Add the goat cheese and stir until it is melted and the mixture looks creamy.

Add the beans, artichokes, tomatoes, herbes de Provence, and salt, and stir to combine. Transfer the contents of the pan to the baking dish.

Mix the bread crumbs, the garlic powder, and the remaining 2 tablespoons of oil in a small bowl. Spread the bread crumbs evenly across the top of the casserole.

Cover the dish with foil and bake for 30 minutes. Remove the foil and bake for 15 more minutes, until the bread crumbs are lightly browned. Cool.

Place about 1½ cups of casserole in each of 8 containers.

STORAGE: Store covered containers in the refrigerator for up to 5 days. Gratin can be frozen for up to 3 months.

Nutrition Info: Total calories: 367; Total fat: 14g; Saturated fat: 5g; Sodium: 624mg; Carbohydrates: 40g; Fiber: 10g; Protein: 1

Steak And Veggies

Servings: 6

Cooking Time: 15 Minutes

Ingredients:

2 lbs baby red potatoes

16 oz broccoli florets

2 tbsp olive oil

3 cloves garlic, minced

1 tsp dried thyme

Kosher salt, to taste

Freshly ground black pepper, to taste

2 lbs (1-inch-thick) top sirloin steak, patted dry

Directions:

Preheat oven to broil

Lightly oil a baking sheet or coat with nonstick spray

In a large pot over high heat, boil salted water, cook the potatoes until parboiled for 12-15 minutes, drain well

Place the potatoes and broccoli in a single layer onto the prepared baking sheet

Add the olive oil, garlic and thyme, season with salt and pepper, to taste and then gently toss to combine

Season the steaks with salt and pepper, to taste, and add to the baking sheet in a single layer

Place it into oven and broil until the steak is browned and charred at the edges, about 4-5 minutes per side for medium-rare, or until the desired doneness

Distribute the steak and veggies among the containers. Store in the fridge for up to 3 days

To Serve: Reheat in the microwave for 1-2 minutes. Top with garlic butter and enjoy

Nutrition Info: Calories:460;Total Fat: 24g;Total Carbs: 24g;Fiber: 2.6g;Protein: 37g

Lentil And Roasted Carrot Salad With Herbs And Feta

Servings: 4

Cooking Time: 25 Minutes

Ingredients:

¾ cup brown or green lentils

3 cups water

1 pound baby carrots, halved on the diagonal

2 teaspoons olive oil, plus 2 tablespoons

½ teaspoon kosher salt, divided

1 teaspoon garlic powder

1 cup packed parsley leaves, chopped

½ cup packed cilantro leaves, chopped

¼ cup packed mint leaves, chopped

½ teaspoon grated lemon zest

4 teaspoons freshly squeezed lemon juice

¼ cup crumbled feta cheese

Directions:

Preheat the oven to 400°F. Line a sheet pan with a silicone baking mat or parchment paper.

Place the lentils and water in a medium saucepan and turn the heat to high. As soon as the water comes to a boil, turn the heat to low and simmer until the lentils are firm yet tender, 10 to minutes (see tip). Drain and cool.

While the lentils are cooking, place the carrots on the sheet pan and toss with 2 teaspoons of oil, ¼ teaspoon of salt, and the garlic powder. Roast the carrots in the oven until firm yet tender, about 20 to 25 minutes. Cool when done.

In a large bowl, mix the cooled lentils, carrots, parsley, cilantro, mint, lemon zest, lemon juice, feta, the remaining 2 tablespoons of oil, and the remaining ¼ teaspoon of salt. Add more lemon juice and/or salt to taste if needed.

Place 1¼ cups of the mixture in each of 4 containers.

STORAGE: Store covered containers in the refrigerator for up to 5 days.

Nutrition Info: Total calories: 2; Total fat: 12g; Saturated fat: 3g; Sodium: 492mg; Carbohydrates: 31g; Fiber: 13g; Protein: 12g

Cinnamon Squash Soup

Servings: 6

Cooking Time: 1 Hour

Ingredients:

1 small butternut squash, peeled and cut up into 1-inch pieces

4 tablespoons extra-virgin olive oil, divided

1 small yellow onion

2 large garlic cloves

1 teaspoon salt, divided

1 pinch black pepper

1 teaspoon dried oregano

2 tablespoons fresh oregano

2 cups low sodium chicken stock

1 cinnamon stick

½ cup canned white kidney beans, drained and rinsed

1 small pear, peeled and cored, chopped up into ½ inch pieces

2 tablespoons walnut pieces

¼ cup Greek yogurt

2 tablespoons freshly chopped parsley

Directions:

Preheat oven to 425 degrees F.

Place squash in bowl and season with a ½ teaspoon of salt and tablespoons of olive oil.

Spread the squash onto a roasting pan and roast for about 25 minutes until tender.

Set aside squash to let cool.

Heat remaining 2 tablespoons of olive oil in a medium-sized pot over medium-high heat.

Add onions and sauté until soft.

Add dried oregano and garlic and sauté for 1 minute and until fragrant.

Add squash, broth, pear, cinnamon stick, pepper, and remaining salt.

Bring mixture to a boil.

Once the boiling point is reached, add walnuts and beans.

Reduce the heat and allow soup to cook for approximately 20 minutes until flavors have blended well.

Remove the cinnamon stick.

Use an immersion blender and blend the entire mixture until smooth.

Add yogurt gradually while whisking to ensure that you are getting a very creamy soup.

Season with some additional salt and pepper if needed.

Garnish with parsley and fresh oregano.

Enjoy!

Nutrition Info: Calories: 197, Total Fat: 11.6 g, Saturated Fat: 1.7 g, Cholesterol: 0 mg, Sodium: 264 mg, Total Carbohydrate: 20.2 g, Dietary Fiber: 7.1 g, Total Sugars: 4.3 g, Protein: 6.1 g, Vitamin D: 0 mcg, Calcium: 103 mg, Iron: 3 mg, Potassium: 425 mg

Creamy Chicken

Servings: 2

Cooking Time: 25 Minutes

Ingredients:

½ small onion, chopped

¼ cup sour cream

Salt and black pepper, to taste

1 tablespoon butter

¼ cup mushrooms

½ pound chicken breasts

Directions:

Heat butter in a skillet and add onions and mushrooms. Sauté for about 5 minutes and add chicken breasts and salt. Secure the lid and cook for about 5 more minutes. Add sour cream and cook for about 3 minutes. Open the lid and dish out in a bowl to serve immediately. Transfer the creamy chicken breasts in a dish and set aside to cool for meal prepping. Divide them in 2 containers and cover their lid. Refrigerate for 2-3 days and reheat in microwave before serving.

Nutrition Info: Calories: 335 ;Carbohydrates: 2.9g;Protein: 34g;Fat: 20.2g;Sugar: 0.8g;Sodium: 154mg

Chicken Drummies With Peach Glaze

Servings: 4

Cooking Time: 25 Minutes

Ingredients:

2 pounds of chicken drummies, remove the skin

15 ounce can of sliced peaches, drain the juice

¼ cup cider vinegar

½ teaspoon paprika

¼ teaspoon black pepper

¼ cup honey

3 garlic cloves

¼ teaspoon sea salt

Directions:

Before you turn your oven on, make sure that one rack is 4 inches below the broiler element.

Set your oven's temperature to 500 degrees Fahrenheit.

Line a large baking sheet with a piece of aluminum foil.

Set a wire cooling rack on top of the foil.

Spray the rack with cooking spray.

Add the honey, peaches, garlic, vinegar, salt, paprika, and pepper into a blender. Mix until smooth.

Set a medium saucepan on top of your stove and set the range temperature to medium heat.

Pour the mixture into the saucepan and bring it to a boil while stirring constantly.

Once the sauce is done, divide it into two small bowls and set one off to the side.

With the second bowl, brush half of the mixture onto the chicken drummies.

Roast the drummies for 10 minutes.

Take the drummies out of the oven and switch to broiler mode.

Brush the drummies with the other half of the sauce from the second bowl.

Again, place the drummies back into the oven and set a timer for 5 minutes.

When the timer goes off, flip the drummies over and broil for another 3 to 4 minutes.

Serve the drummies with the reserved sauce and enjoy!

Nutrition Info: calories: 291, fats: 5 grams, carbohydrates: 33 grams, protein: 30 grams.

Berry Compote With Orange Mint Infusion

Servings: 8

Cooking Time: 20 Minutes

Ingredients:

½ cup water

3 orange pekoe tea bags

3 sprigs of fresh mint

1 cup fresh strawberries, hulled and halved lengthwise

1 cup fresh golden raspberries

1 cup fresh red raspberries

1 cup fresh blueberries

1 cup fresh blackberries

1 cup fresh sweet cherries, pitted and halved

1-milliliter bottle of Sauvignon Blanc

2/3 cup sugar

½ cup pomegranate juice

1 teaspoon vanilla

fresh mint sprigs

Directions:

In a small saucepan, bring water to a boil and add tea bags and 3 mint sprigs.

Stir well, cover, remove from heat, and allow to stand for 10 minutes.

In a large bowl, add strawberries, red raspberries, golden raspberries, blueberries, blackberries, and cherries. Put to the side.

In a medium-sized saucepan, and add the wine, sugar, and pomegranate juice.

Pour the infusion (tea mixture) through a fine-mesh sieve and into the pan with wine.

Squeeze the bags to release the liquid, and then discard bags and mint springs.

Cook well until the sugar has completely dissolved; remove from heat.

Stir in vanilla and allow to chill for 2 hours.

Pour the mix over the fruits.

Garnish with mint sprigs and serve.

Enjoy!

Nutrition Info: Calories: 119, Total Fat: 0.3 g, Saturated Fat: 0 g, Cholesterol: 0 mg, Sodium: 3 mg, Total Carbohydrate: 31.6 g, Dietary Fiber: 5 g, Total Sugars: 26.2 g, Protein: 1.2 g, Vitamin D: 0 mcg, Calcium: 28 mg, Iron: 1 mg, Potassium: 158 mg

Quinoa Bruschetta Salad

Servings: 5

Cooking Time: 15 Minutes

Ingredients:

2 cups water

1 cup uncooked quinoa

1 (10-ounce) container cherry tomatoes, quartered

1 teaspoon chopped garlic

1¼ cups thinly sliced scallions, white and green parts (1 small bunch)

1 (8-ounce) container fresh whole-milk mozzarella balls (ciliegine), quartered

2 tablespoons balsamic vinegar

2 tablespoons olive oil

½ teaspoon kosher salt

½ cup fresh basil leaves, chiffonaded (cut into strips)

Directions:

Place the water and quinoa in a saucepan and bring to a boil. Cover, turn the heat to low, and simmer for minutes.

While the quinoa is cooking, place the tomatoes, garlic, scallions, mozzarella, vinegar, and oil in a large mixing bowl. Stir to combine.

Once the quinoa is cool, add it to the tomato mixture along with the salt and basil. Mix to combine.

Place 1⅓ cups of the mixture in each of 5 containers and refrigerate. Serve at room temperature.

STORAGE: Store covered containers in the refrigerator for up to days.

Nutrition Info: Total calories: 323; Total fat: 1; Saturated fat: 6g; Sodium: 317mg; Carbohydrates: 30g; Fiber: 4g; Protein: 14g

Zesty Lemon Parmesan Chicken And Zucchini Noodles

Servings: 2

Cooking Time: 15 Minutes

Ingredients:

2 packages Frozen zucchini noodle Spirals

1-1/2 lbs. boneless skinless chicken breast, cut into bite-sized pieces

1 tsp fine sea salt

2 tsp dried oregano

1/2 tsp ground black pepper

4 garlic cloves, minced

2 tbsp vegan butter

2 tsp lemon zest

2 tsp oil

1/3 cup parmesan

2/3 cup broth

Lemon slices, for garnish

Parsley, for garnish

Directions:

Cook zucchini noodles according to package instructions, drain well

In a large skillet over medium heat, add the oil

Season chicken with salt and pepper, brown chicken pieces, for about 4 minutes per side depending on the thickness, or until cooked through – Work in cook in batches if necessary

Transfer the chicken to a pan

In the same skillet, add in the garlic, and cook until fragrant about 30 seconds

Add in the butter, oregano and lemon zest, pour in chicken broth to deglaze making sure to scrape up all the browned bits stuck to the bottom of the pan

Turn the heat up to medium-high, bring sauce and chicken up to a boil, immediately lower the heat and stir in the parmesan cheese

Place the chicken back in pan and allow it to gently simmer for 3-4 minutes, or until sauce has slightly reduced and thickened up

Taste and adjust seasoning, allow the noodles to cool completely

Distribute among the containers, store for 2-3 days

To Serve: Reheat in the microwave for 1-2 minutes or until heated through. Garnish with the fresh parsley and lemon slices and enjoy!

Nutrition Info: Calories:633;Carbs: 4g;Total Fat: 35g;Protein: 70g

Three Citrus Sauce Scallops

Servings: 4

Cooking Time: 15 Minutes

Ingredients:

2 teaspoons extra virgin olive oil

1 shallot, minced

20 sea scallops, cleaned

1 tablespoon lemon zest

2 teaspoons orange zest

1 teaspoon lime zest

1 tablespoon fresh basil, chopped

½ cup freshly squeezed lemon juice

2 tablespoons honey

1 tablespoon plain Greek yogurt

Pinch of sea salt

Directions:

Take a large skillet and place it over medium-high heat

Add olive oil and heat it up

Add shallots and Saute for 1 minute

Add scallops in the skillet and sear for 5 minutes, turning once

Move scallops to edge and stir in lemon, orange, lime zest, basil, orange juice and lemon juice

Simmer the sauce for 3 minutes

Whisk in honey, yogurt and salt

Cook for 4 minutes and coat the scallops in the sauce

Serve and enjoy!

Meal Prep/Storage Options: Store in airtight containers in your fridge for 1-2 days.

Nutrition Info: Calories: 207;Fat: 4g;Carbohydrates: 17g;Protein: 26g

Steamed Mussels Topped With Wine Sauce

Servings: 4

Cooking Time: 15 Minutes

Ingredients:

2 pounds mussels

1 tablespoon extra virgin olive oil

1 cup sliced onion

1 cup dry white wine

¼ teaspoon ground black pepper

¼ teaspoon sea salt

3 sliced cloves of garlic

2 lemon slices

Optional: lemon wedges for serving

Directions:

Set a large colander in the sink and turn your water to cold.

Run water over the mussels, but do not let them sit in the water.

If you notice any shells that are not tightly sealed or are cracked, you need to discard them. All shells need to be closed tightly.

Turn off the water and leave the mussels in the colander.

Set a large skillet on your stovetop and turn your range heat to medium-high.

Pour the olive oil into the skillet and allow it to heat up before you add the onion.

Saute the onion for 2 to 3 minutes.

Combine the garlic and cook the mixture for another minute while stirring continuously.

Pour in the wine, pepper, lemon slices, and salt. Stir the ingredients as you bring them to a boil.

Add the mussels and place the lid on the skillet.

Cook the mixture for 3 to 4 minutes or until the shells begin to open on the mussels. It will help to gently pick up the skillet and shake it a couple of times when the mussels are cooking.

If you notice any shells that did not open, use a spoon and discard them.

Scoop the mussels into a serving bowl and pour the mixture over the top.

If you have lemon wedges, place them on the top of the steamed mussels before serving. Enjoy!

Nutrition Info: calories: 222, fats: 7 grams, carbohydrates: 11 grams, protein: 18 grams.

Spice Potato Soup

Servings: 4-6

Cooking Time: 30 Minutes

Ingredients:

2 tablespoons extra virgin olive oil

1 large onion, chopped

2 garlic cloves, crushed

1 pound sweet potatoes, peeled and cut into medium pieces

½ teaspoon ground cumin

¼ teaspoon ground chili

½ teaspoon ground coriander

¼ teaspoon ground cinnamon

¼ teaspoon salt

2 cups chicken stock

¼ cup of low-fat crème Fraiche

2 tablespoons freshly chopped parsley

Coriander

Directions:

Heat olive oil in a large pan over medium-high heat.

Add onions and sauté until slightly browned.

Reduce heat to medium, add garlic, and keep cooking for 2-minutes more.

Add sweet potatoes and sauté for 3-minutes.

Add the remaining spices and season with salt.

Cook for 2 minutes.

Add stock, turn the heat up, and bring the mixture to a boil, stirring occasionally.

Cover and lower heat to a slow simmer.

Cook for 20 minutes until the potatoes are tender.

Remove the pan from the heat.

Take an immersion blender and puree the whole mixture.

Add a bit of water if the soup is too thick.

Check the soup for seasoning.

Ladle the soup into your jars.

Give a swirl of crème Fraiche.

Sprinkle with chopped parsley.

Enjoy!

Nutrition Info: Calories: 176, Total Fat: 8.4 g, Saturated Fat: 0.8 g, Cholesterol: 0 mg, Sodium: 362 mg, Total Carbohydrate: 24.3 g, Dietary Fiber: 3.8 g, Total Sugars: 1.7 g, Protein: 2 g, Vitamin D: 0 mcg, Calcium: 30 mg, Iron: 1 mg, Potassium: 675 mg

Spicy Cajun Shrimp

Servings: 2

Cooking Time: 50 Minutes

Ingredients:

3 cloves garlic, crushed

4 tablespoons butter, divided

2 large zucchini, spiraled

1 red pepper, sliced

1 onion, sliced

20-30 jumbo shrimp

1 teaspoon paprika

dash cayenne pepper

½ teaspoon of sea salt

dash red pepper flakes

1 teaspoon garlic powder

1 teaspoon onion powder

Directions:

Pass the zucchini through a spiralizer.

Combine the Ingredients: listed under Cajun Seasoning above.

Add oil and 2 tablespoons of butter to a pan and allow to heat up over medium heat.

Add onion and red pepper and sauté for minutes.

Add shrimp and cook well.

Place the remaining 2 tablespoons of butter in another pan and allow it to melt over medium heat.

Add zucchini noodles and sauté for 3 minutes.

Transfer the noodles to a container.

Top with the prepared Cajun shrimp and veggie mix.

Season with salt and enjoy!

Nutrition Info: Calories: 734, Total Fat: 24.2 g, Saturated Fat: 14.7 g, Cholesterol: 12mg, Sodium: 6703 mg, Total Carbohydrate: 29.1 g, Dietary Fiber: 7.1 g, Total Sugars: 24.9 g, Protein: 106.8 g, Vitamin D: 16 mcg, Calcium: 694 mg, Iron: 6 mg, Potassium: 1229 mg

Pan-seared Salmon

Servings: 4

Cooking Time: 20 Minutes

Ingredients:

Salmon fillets (4 @ 6 oz. each)

Olive oil (2 tbsp.)

Capers (2 tbsp.)

Pepper & salt (.125 tsp. each)

Lemon (4 slices)

Directions:

Warm a heavy skillet for about three minutes using the medium heat temperature setting.

Lightly spritz the salmon with oil. Arrange them in the pan and increase the temperature setting to high.

Sear for approximately three minutes. Sprinkle with the salt, pepper, and capers.

Flip the salmon over and continue cooking for five minutes or until browned the way you like it.

Garnish with lemon slices and serve.

Nutrition Info: Calories: 371;Protein: 33.7 grams; Fat: 25.1 grams

Pasta Faggioli Soup

Servings: 8

Cooking Time: 1 Hour

Ingredients:

1 28-ounce can diced tomatoes

1 14-ounce can great northern beans, undrained

14 ounces spinach, chopped and drained

1 14-ounce can tomato sauce

3 cups chicken broth

1 tablespoon garlic, minced

8 slices bacon, cooked crisp, crumbled

1 tablespoon dried parsley

1 teaspoon garlic powder

1½ teaspoons salt

½ teaspoon ground black pepper

½ teaspoon dried basil

½ pound seashell pasta

3 cups water

Directions:

Take a large stockpot and add the diced tomatoes, spinach, beans, chicken broth, tomato sauce, water, bacon, garlic, parsley, garlic powder, pepper, salt, and basil.

Put it over medium-high heat and bring the mixture to a boil.

Immediately reduce the heat to low and simmer for 40 minutes, covered.

Add pasta and cook uncovered for about 10 minutes until al dente.

Ladle the soup into serving bowls.

Sprinkle some cheese on top.

Enjoy!

Nutrition Info: Calories: 23 Total Fat: 2.3 g, Saturated Fat: 0.7 g, Cholesterol: 2 mg, Sodium: 2232 mg, Total Carbohydrate: 40.6 g, Dietary Fiber: 13.1 g, Total Sugars: 6.4 g, Protein: 16.3 g, Vitamin D: 0 mcg, Calcium: 160 mg, Iron: 5 mg, Potassium: 1455 mg

Fattoush Salad

Servings: 4

Cooking Time: 10 Minutes

Ingredients:

2 loaves pita bread

3 tablespoons extra virgin olive oil

½ teaspoon of sumac

salt

pepper

1 heart romaine lettuce, chopped

1 English cucumber, chopped

5 Roma tomatoes, chopped

5 green onions, chopped

5 radishes, stems removed, thinly sliced

2 cups fresh parsley leaves, stems removed, chopped

1 cup fresh mint leaves, chopped

lime juice, 1½ limes

1/3 bottle extra virgin olive oil

salt

pepper

1 teaspoon ground sumac

¼ teaspoon ground cinnamon

scant ¼ teaspoon ground allspice

Directions:

Toast pita bread until crisp but not browned.

Heat 3 tablespoons of olive oil in a large pan over medium heat.

Break the toasted pita into pieces and add them to the oil.

Fry pita bread until browned, making sure to toss them from time to time.

Add salt, ½ a teaspoon of sumac, and pepper.

Remove the pita from the heat and place on a paper towel to drain.

In a large mixing bowl, combine lettuce, tomatoes, cucumber, green onions, parsley, and radish.

Before serving, make the lime vinaigrette by mixing all Ingredients: listed above under vinaigrette in a separate bowl.

Pour the vinaigrette over the Ingredients: in the other bowl and gently toss.

Add pita chips on top and the remaining sumac.

Give it a final toss and enjoy!

Nutrition Info: Calories: 200, Total Fat: 11.5 g, Saturated Fat: 1.7 g, Cholesterol: 0 mg, Sodium: 113 mg, Total Carbohydrate: 23.5 g, Dietary Fiber: 5.8 g, Total Sugars: 6.6 g, Protein: 5.2 g, Vitamin D: 0 mcg, Calcium: 145 mg, Iron: 6 mg, Potassium: 852 mg

Roast Chicken

Servings: 6

Cooking Time: 1 – 1 ½ Hour

Ingredients:

fresh orange juice, 1 large orange

¼ cup Dijon mustard

¼ cup olive oil

4 teaspoons dried Greek oregano

salt

ground black pepper

12 potatoes, peeled and cubed

5 garlic cloves, minced

1 whole chicken

Directions:

Preheat oven to 375 degrees F.

Take a bowl and whisk in orange juice, Greek oregano, Dijon mustard, salt, and pepper. Mix well.

Add potatoes to the bowl and coat them thoroughly.

Transfer the potatoes to a large baking dish, leaving remaining juice in a bowl.

Stuff the garlic cloves into your chicken (under the skin).

Place the chicken into the bowl with the remaining juice and coat it thoroughly.

Transfer chicken to the baking dish, placing it on top of the potatoes.

Pour any extra juice on top of chicken and potatoes.

Bake uncovered until the thickest part of the chicken registers 160 degrees F, and the juices run clear, anywhere from 60 – minutes.

Remove the chicken and cover it with doubled aluminum foil.

Allow it to rest for 10 minutes.

Slice, spread over containers and enjoy!

Nutrition Info: Calories: 1080, Total Fat: 36.4 g, Saturated Fat: 8.8 g, Cholesterol: 325 mg, Sodium: 458 mg, Total Carbohydrate: 70.5 g, Dietary Fiber: 11.1 g, Total Sugars: 6.3 g, Protein: 16 g, Vitamin D: 0 mcg, Calcium: 120 mg, Iron: 7 mg, Potassium: 2691 mg

Chicken Eggplant

Servings: 5

Cooking Time: 40 Minutes

Ingredients:

3 pieces of eggplants, peeled and cut up lengthwise into ½ inch slices

3 tablespoons olive oil

6 skinless and boneless chicken breast halves, diced

1 onion, diced

2 tablespoons tomato paste

½ cup water

2 teaspoons dried oregano

Salt

Pepper

Directions:

Place the eggplant strips in a large pot filled with lightly salted water.

Allow them to soak for 30 minutes.

Remove the eggplant from the pot and brush thoroughly with olive oil.

Heat a skillet over medium heat.

Add eggplant and sauté for a few minutes.

Transfer the sautéed eggplant to a baking dish.

Heat a large skillet over medium heat.

Add chicken, onion, and sauté.

Stir in water and tomato paste.

Reduce heat to low, cover, and simmer for minutes.

Preheat oven to 400 degrees F.

Pour the chicken tomato mix over your eggplant.

Season with oregano, pepper, and salt.

Cover with aluminum foil and bake for 20 minutes.

Cool, place to containers and chill.

Nutrition Info: Calories: 319, Total Fat: 11.3 g, Saturated Fat: 1.2 g, Cholesterol: 117 mg, Sodium: 143 mg, Total Carbohydrate: 7.2 g, Dietary Fiber: 3.1 g, Total Sugars: 3.5 g, Protein: 48 g, Vitamin D: 0 mcg, Calcium: 22 mg, Iron: 2 mg, Potassium: 244 mg

Grilled Steak

Servings: 2

Cooking Time: 15 Minutes

Ingredients:

¼ cup unsalted butter

2 garlic cloves, minced

¾ pound beef top sirloin steaks

¾ teaspoon dried rosemary, crushed

2 oz. parmesan cheese, shredded

Salt and black pepper, to taste

Directions:

Preheat the grill and grease it. Season the sirloin steaks with salt and black pepper. Transfer the steaks on the grill and cook for about 5 minutes on each side. Dish out the steaks in plates and keep aside. Meanwhile, put butter and garlic in a pan and heat until melted. Pour it on the steaks and serve hot. Divide the steaks in 2 containers and refrigerate for about 3 days for meal prepping purpose. Reheat in microwave before serving.

Nutrition Info: Calories: 3 ; Carbohydrates: 1.5g ;Protein: 41.4g;Fat: 23.6g;Sugar: 0g;Sodium: 352mg

Beef And Veggie Lasagna

Servings: 10

Cooking Time: 1 Hour 10 Minutes

Ingredients:

3 teaspoons olive oil, divided

1 medium zucchini, quartered lengthwise and chopped (about 1⅓ cups)

3 cups packed baby spinach

1 cup chopped yellow onion

1 teaspoon chopped garlic

8 ounces button or cremini mushrooms, finely chopped

1 cup shredded carrots

8 ounces lean (90/10) ground beef

½ cup dry red wine

1 (28-ounce) can low-sodium or no-salt-added crushed tomatoes

1 (15-ounce) can tomato sauce

¼ teaspoon kosher salt

1 (16-ounce) container low-fat (2%) cottage cheese

1 large egg

3 tablespoons grated Parmesan cheese

2 cups shredded part-skim mozzarella cheese, divided

½ cup fresh basil leaves, chopped

1 (9-ounce) box oven-ready lasagna noodles

Directions:

Preheat the oven to 375°F.

Heat 1 teaspoon of oil in a 1inch skillet over medium-high heat. When the oil is shimmering, add the zucchini and cook for 2 minutes. Add the spinach and continue to cook for 1 more minute. Remove the veggies to a plate.

In the same skillet, heat the remaining 2 teaspoons of oil over medium-high heat. When the oil is hot, add the onion and garlic and cook for 2 minutes. Add the mushrooms and carrots and cook for 4 more minutes. Add the ground beef and continue cooking for 4 more minutes, until the meat has browned. Add the wine and cook for 1 minute. Add the crushed tomatoes, tomato sauce, and salt, stir, and turn off the heat.

In a large mixing bowl, combine the cottage cheese, egg, and Parmesan, ½ cup of shredded cheese, and the basil.

Ladle 2 cups of sauce on the bottom of a 9-by-13-inch glass or ceramic baking dish. Place 4 noodles side by side in the pan. Layer 1 cup of sauce, half of the veggies, and half of the cottage cheese. Repeat with 4 more noodles, 1 cup of sauce, the remaining half of the veggies, and the remaining half of the cottage cheese. Top with 4 more noodles, the remainder of the sauce, and the remaining 1½ cups of shredded cheese.

Cover the pan with foil, trying not to touch the foil to the cheese, and bake for 40 minutes. Remove the foil and bake for 10 to 15 more minutes, until the cheese starts to brown.

When the lasagna cools, cut it into 10 pieces and place 1 piece in each of 10 containers.

STORAGE: Store covered containers in the refrigerator for up to 5 days. Cooked lasagna freezes well and can last for up to 3 months.

Nutrition Info: Total calories: 321; Total fat: 11g; Saturated fat: 4g; Sodium: 680mg; Carbohydrates: 34g; Fiber: 5g; Protein: 24g

Greek Shrimp And Farro Bowls

Servings: 4

Cooking Time: 20 Minutes

Ingredients:

1 lb peeled and deveined shrimp

3 Tbsp. extra virgin olive oil

2 cloves garlic, minced

2 bell peppers, sliced thick

2 medium-sized zucchinis, sliced into thin rounds

pint cherry tomatoes, halved

¼ cup thinly sliced green or black olives

4 Tbsp. 2% reduced-fat plain Greek yogurt

Juice of 1 lemon

2 tsp fresh chopped dill

1 Tbsp. fresh chopped oregano

½ tsp smoked paprika

½ tsp sea salt

¼ tsp black pepper

1 cup dry farro

Directions:

In a bowl, add the olive oil, garlic, lemon, dill, oregano, paprika, salt, and pepper, whisk to combine

Pour 3/4 the amount of marinade over shrimp, toss to coat and all to stand 10 minutes

Reserve the rest of the marinade for later

Cook the farro according to package instructions in water or chicken stock

In a grill pan or nonstick skillet over medium heat, add the olive

Once heated, add shrimp, cook for 2-3 minutes per side, until no longer pink, then transfer to a plate

Working in batches, cook bell pepper, zucchinis, and cherry tomatoes to the grill pan or skillet, cook for 5-6 minutes, until softened

allow the dish to cool completely

Distribute the farro among the containers, evenly add the shrimp, grilled vegetables, olives, and tomatoes, store for 2 days

To Serve: Reheat in the microwave for 1-2 minutes or until heated through. Drizzle the reserved marinade over top. Top each bowl with 1 tbsp Greek yogurt and extra lemon juice, if desired

Nutrition Info: Calories:428;Carbs: 45g;Total Fat: 13g;Protein: 34g

Asparagus Salmon Fillets

Servings: 2

Cooking Time: 30 Minutes

Ingredients:

1 teaspoon olive oil

4 asparagus stalks

2 salmon fillets

¼ cup butter

¼ cup champagne

Salt and freshly ground black pepper, to taste

Directions:

Preheat the oven to 355 degrees F and grease a baking dish.

Put all the ingredients in a bowl and mix well.

Put this mixture in the baking dish and transfer it in the oven.

Bake for about 20 minutes and dish out.

Place the salmon fillets in a dish and keep aside to cool for meal prepping. Divide it into 2 containers and close the lid. Refrigerate for 1 day and reheat in microwave before serving.

Nutrition Info: Calories: 475 ;Carbohydrates: 1.1g;Protein: 35.2g;Fat: 38g;Sugar: 0.5g;Sodium: 242mg

Grilled Calamari With Berries

Servings: 4
Cooking Time: 5 Minutes

Ingredients:

¼ cup olive oil

¼ cup extra virgin olive oil

1 thinly sliced apple

¾ cup blueberries

¼ cup sliced almonds

1 ½ pounds calamari tube

¼ cup dried cranberries

6 cups spinach

2 tablespoons apple cider vinegar

1 tablespoon lemon juice

Sea salt and pepper to your liking

Directions:

Start by making the vinaigrette. Combine apple cider vinegar, lemon juice, extra virgin olive oil, sea salt, and pepper. Whisk well and set aside.

Set your grill to medium heat.

In a separate bowl, add the calamari tube and mix with salt, pepper, and olive oil.

Set the calamari on the grill and cook both sides for 2 to 3 minutes.

In another bowl, mix the salad by adding the spinach, cranberries, almonds, blueberries, and apples. Toss to mix.

Set the cooked calamari onto a cutting board and let it cool for a few minutes. Cut them into ¼-inch thick rings and then toss them into the salad bowl.

Sprinkle the vinaigrette sauce onto the salad. Toss to mix the ingredients and enjoy!

Nutrition Info: calories: 567, fats: 24.4 grams, carbohydrates: 30 grams, protein: 55 grams.

Italian Sausage And Veggie Pizza Pasta

Servings: 8

Cooking Time: 30 Minutes

Ingredients:

1 tsp olive oil

1 (2.25 oz) can of sliced black olives

1 (28 oz) can of tomato sauce

1 (16 oz) box penne pasta

3 cups water

3 sweet Italian sausage links, casings removed, around 1 lb of sausage

1 cup sliced onions

1 cup sliced green bell pepper

2-3 garlic cloves, minced or pressed

8 oz. sliced mushrooms

1/2 cup Pepperoni, cut in half and then each half cut into thirds + a few extra whole pieces for topping

1/2 tsp Italian seasoning

1/2 tsp salt

Salt, to taste

Pepper to taste

2 cups shredded mozzarella cheese, divided

Garnish:

Chopped fresh parsley and Romano cheese

Directions:

In a deep heavy-bottom, oven-safe pot over medium heat, add the oil

Once heated, add in the sausage and break it up with a wooden spoon

Then add in the onions, peppers, garlic and mushrooms, stir to combine, season with salt and pepper to taste. Sauté until the sausage crumbles have browned, stirring frequently for around 10 minutes

Add in the pepperoni and olives to the pan, sauté for 1-2 minutes. Then add in the sauce, water, Italian seasoning, salt and pasta to the pan, stir to combine

Bring the pot to a boil

Once boiling, reduce the heat to medium low, cover and allow to simmer for 10 minutes, stirring occasionally

Remove the cover and continue to simmer for 3-5 minutes, stirring occasionally

Stir in 1/2 cup of shredded Mozzarella cheese, sprinkle the remaining cheese on top

Arrange a few more whole pepperonis on top of the cheese, broil for a few minutes until the cheese is bubbling and melted

Top with the parsley and Romano cheese

Allow to cool and distribute the pasta evenly among the containers. Store in the fridge for 3-4 days or in the freezer for 2 weeks.

To Serve: Reheat in the oven at 375 degrees for 1-2 minutes or until heated through.

Recipe Note: If you would like it to be spicy, you can also use hot Italian sausage.

Nutrition Info: Calories:450;Total Fat: 21.9g;Total Carbs: 22g;Fiber: 5g;Protein: 43g

Baked Chicken Thighs With Lemon, Olives, And Brussels Sprouts

Servings: 4

Cooking Time: 40 Minutes

Ingredients:

2 tablespoons olive oil, divided

1 pound Brussels sprouts, stemmed and halved (quartered if the sprouts are extra large)

1 pound boneless, skinless chicken thighs

2 teaspoons chopped garlic

1 teaspoon dried oregano

½ teaspoon kosher salt

3 tablespoons freshly squeezed lemon juice

½ cup pitted kalamata olives

Directions:

Preheat the oven to 350°F.

Spread 1 tablespoon of oil over the bottom of a 13-by-9-inch glass or ceramic baking dish. Add the Brussels sprouts to the pan and spread out evenly. Place the chicken on top of the sprouts and rub the garlic and oregano into the top of the chicken.

Sprinkle the salt, the remaining 1 tablespoon of oil, the lemon juice, and the olives over the contents of the pan.

Cover the pan with aluminum foil and bake for 20 minutes. Remove the foil and bake uncovered for 20 more minutes. Cool.

Place one quarter of the chicken and ¾ cup of Brussels sprouts in each of 4 containers. Drizzle any remaining juices from the pan over the chicken.

STORAGE: Store covered containers in the refrigerator for 5 days.

Nutrition Info: Total calories: 28 Total fat: 18g; Saturated fat: 3g; Sodium: 737mg; Carbohydrates: 14g; Fiber: 5g; Protein: 20g

Slow Cooker Lamb, Herb, And Bean Stew

Servings: 4

Cooking Time: 15 Minutes

Ingredients:

3 bunches of parsley (about 6 packed cups of leaves)

1 large bunch cilantro (about 1½ packed cups of leaves)

1 bunch scallions, sliced (both white and green parts, about 1¼ cups)

1 pound leg of lamb, fat trimmed, cut into 1-inch pieces

2 tablespoons olive oil, divided

1 medium onion, chopped

2 teaspoons chopped garlic

2 teaspoons turmeric

¾ teaspoon kosher salt

2 tablespoons tomato paste

2½ cups low-sodium chicken broth

2 (15.5-ounce) cans low-sodium kidney beans, drained and rinsed

2 tablespoons freshly squeezed lemon juice

Directions:

Finely chop the parsley leaves, cilantro leaves, and scallions with a knife, or pulse in the food processor until finely chopped but not puréed. With this amount of herbs, you'll need to pulse in two batches.

Pat the lamb cubes with a paper towel. Heat a 1inch skillet over medium-high heat and add 1 tablespoon of oil. Once the oil is shimmering, add the lamb and brown for 5 minutes, flipping after 3 minutes. Place the lamb in the slow cooker.

Turn the heat down to medium and add the remaining 1 tablespoon of oil to the skillet. Once the oil is hot, add the onions and garlic and sauté for minutes. Add the turmeric, salt, and tomato paste and continue to cook for 2 more minutes, stirring frequently.

Add the chopped parsley, cilantro, and scallions. Sauté for 5 minutes, stirring occasionally.

While the herbs are cooking, add the broth, beans, and lemon juice to the slow cooker. Add the herb mixture when it's done cooking on the stove. Turn the slow cooker to the low setting and cook for 8 hours.

Taste and add more salt and/or lemon juice if needed. Cool.

Scoop 2 cups of stew into each of 4 containers.

STORAGE: Store covered containers in the refrigerator for up to 5 days. Stew can be frozen for up to 4 months.

Nutrition Info: Total calories: 486; Total fat: 15g; Saturated fat: 5g; Sodium: 6mg; Carbohydrates: 51g; Fiber: 15g; Protein: 41g

Holiday Chicken Salad

Servings: 2

Cooking Time: 25 Minutes

Ingredients:

1 celery stalk, chopped

1½ cups cooked grass-fed chicken, chopped

¼ cup fresh cranberries

¼ cup sour cream

½ apple, chopped

¼ yellow onion, chopped

1/8 cup almonds, toasted and chopped

2-ounce feta cheese, crumbled

¼ cup avocado mayonnaise

Salt and black pepper, to taste

Directions:

Stir together all the ingredients in a bowl except almonds and cheese. Top with almonds and cheese to serve. Meal Prep Tip: Don't add almonds and cheese in the salad if you want to store the salad. Cover with a plastic wrap and refrigerate to serve.

Nutrition Info: Calories: 336 ;Carbohydrates: 8.8g;Protein: 25g;Fat: 23.2g ;Sugar: 5.4g;Sodium: 383mg

Costa Brava Chicken

Servings: 4

Cooking Time: 35 Minutes

Ingredients:

1 20-ounce can pineapple chunks

10 skinless and boneless chicken breast halves

1 tablespoon vegetable oil

1 teaspoon ground cumin

1 teaspoon ground cinnamon

2garlic cloves, minced

1 onion, quartered

1 14-ounce can stewed tomatoes

2 cups black olives

½ cup salsa

2 tablespoons water

1 red bell pepper, thinly sliced

Salt

Directions:

Drain the pineapple chunks, but be sure to reserve the juice.

Sprinkle pineapples with salt.

Heat oil in a large frying pan over medium heat.

Add the chicken and cook until brown.

Combine the cinnamon and cumin and sprinkle over the chicken.
Add garlic and onion and cook until the onions are tender.
Add reserved pineapple juices, olives, tomatoes, and salsa.
Reduce heat, cover, and allow to simmer for 25 minutes.
Combine the cornstarch and water in a bowl.
Add the cornstarch mixture to the pan and stir.
Add the bell pepper and simmer for a little longer until the sauce bubbles and thickens.
Stir in pineapple chunks until thoroughly heated.
Enjoy!

Nutrition Info: Calories: 651, Total Fat: 16.5 g, Saturated Fat: 1.7 g, Cholesterol: 228 mg, Sodium: 1053 mg, Total Carbohydrate: 34.7 g, Dietary Fiber: 7.2 g, Total Sugars: 20.3 g, Protein: 94.5 g, Vitamin D: 0 mcg, Calcium: 118 mg, Iron: 6 mg, Potassium: 606 mg

One Skillet Greek Lemon Chicken And Rice

Servings: 5

Cooking Time: 45 Minutes

Ingredients:

Marinade:

2 tsp dried oregano

1 tsp dried minced onion

4-5 cloves garlic, minced

Zest of 1 lemon

1/2 tsp kosher salt

1/2 tsp black pepper

1-2 Tbsp olive oil to make a loose paste

5 bone-in, skin on chicken thighs

Rice:

1 1/2 Tbsp olive oil

1 large yellow onion, peeled and diced

1 cup dry long-grain white rice (NOT minute or quick cooking varieties)

2 cups chicken stock

1 1/4 tsp dried oregano

5 cloves garlic, minced

3/4 tsp kosher salt

1/2 tsp black pepper

Lemon slices, optional

Fresh minced parsley, for garnish

Extra lemon zest, for garnish

Directions:

In a large resealable plastic bag, add the oregano, dried minced onion, garlic, lemon zest, salt, black pepper, and olive oil, massage to combine

Add chicken thighs, and then turn/massage to coat, refrigerate 15 minutes or overnight

Preheat oven to 0 F degrees

In a large cast iron or heavy oven safe skillet over medium-high heat, add 1 1/2 Tbsp olive oil to

Remove the chicken thighs from the refrigerator, shake off the excess marinade and add chicken thighs, skin side down, to pan, cook 4-minutes per side

Transfer to a plate and wipe the skillet lightly with a paper towel to remove any burnt bits, reserving chicken grease in pan.

Lower the heat to medium and add onion to pan, cook 3-4 minutes, until softened and slightly charred. Add in garlic and cook 1 minute

Then add in the rice, oregano, salt and pepper, stir together and cook for 1 minute

Pour in chicken stock, turn the temperature up to medium-high, bring to a simmer

Once simmering, place the chicken thighs on top of the rice mixture, push down gently

Cover with lid or foil, and bake 35 minutes

Uncover, return to oven and bake an additional 10-15 minutes, until liquid is removed, the rice is tender, and chicken is cooked through

Allow the rice and chicken to cool

Distribute among the containers, store in fridge for 2-3 days

To serve: Reheat in the microwave for 1 minute to 2 minutes or cooked through. Garnish with lemon zest and parsley, and serve!

Nutrition Info: Calories:325;Carbs: 35g;Total Fat: 11g;Protein: 21g

Trout With Wilted Greens

Servings: 4

Cooking Time: 15 Minutes

Ingredients:

2 teaspoons extra virgin olive oil

2 cups kale, chopped

2 cups Swiss chard, chopped

½ sweet onion, thinly sliced

4 (5 ounce boneless skin-on trout fillets)

Juice of 1 lemon

Sea salt

Freshly ground pepper

Zest of 1 lemon

Directions:

Pre-heat your oven to 375-degree Fahrenheit

Lightly grease a 9 by 13-inch baking dish with olive oil

Arrange the kale, Swiss chard, onion in a dish

Top greens with fish, skin side up and drizzle with olive oil and lemon juice

Season fish with salt and pepper

Bake for 15 minutes until fish flakes

Sprinkle zest

Serve and enjoy!

Meal Prep/Storage Options: Store in airtight containers in your fridge for 1-3 days.

Nutrition Info: Calories: 315;Fat: 14g;Carbohydrates: 6g;Protein: 39g

One Skillet Chicken In Roasted Red Pepper Sauce

Servings: 4

Cooking Time: 20 Minutes

Ingredients:

4-6 boneless skinless chicken thighs or breasts

2/3 cup chopped roasted red peppers (see note)

2 tsp Italian seasoning, divided

4 tbsp oil

1 tbsp minced garlic

1/2 tsp salt

1/4 tsp black pepper

1 cup heavy cream

2 tbsp crumbled feta cheese, optional

Thinly sliced fresh basil, optional

Directions:

In a blender or food processer, combine the roasted red peppers, tsp Italian seasoning, oil, garlic, salt, and pepper, pulse until smooth.

In a large skillet over medium heat, add the olive oil and season chicken with remaining 1 tsp Italian seasoning. Cook chicken for

6-8 minutes on each side, or until cooked through and lightly browned on the outside. Then transfer to a plate and cover

Add the red pepper mixture to the pan, stir over medium heat 2-minutes, or until heated throughout. Add the heavy cream, stir until mixture is thick and creamy

Add chicken, toss in the sauce to coat

allow the dish to cool completely

Distribute among the containers, store for 2-3 days

To Serve: Reheat in the microwave for 1-2 minutes or until heated through. Garnish with crumbled feta cheese and fresh basil. Serve with your favorite grain.

Recipe Notes: You can purchase jarred roasted red peppers at most grocery stores around the olives.

Nutrition Info: Calories:655;Carbs: 12g;Total Fat: 25g;Protein: 8

Mediterranean Minestrone Soup

Servings: 4

Cooking Time: 40 Minutes

Ingredients:

1 large onion, finely chopped

4 cups vegetable stock

4 cloves crushed garlic

1 ounce chopped carrots

4 ounces chopped red bell pepper

4 ounces chopped celery (keep leaves)

1 16-ounce can diced tomatoes

1 16-ounce can white beans

4 ounces fresh spinach, chopped

4 ounces multi-colored pasta

2 ounces grated parmesan

2 tablespoons olive oil

bunch of chopped parsley

1 teaspoon dried oregano

salt

pepper

4 ounces salami, finely sliced (if desired)

Directions:

Heat oil in a pan over medium heat.

Add chopped onions, red pepper, carrots, and celery.

Saute for about 10 minutes until tender.

Add garlic and cook on low heat for 2 minutes more.

Add your stock and tomatoes and cook for an additional 10 minutes.

Add pasta and cook for 15 minutes more until al dente.

Taste / check your seasoning; add salt and pepper as needed.

Add parsley, beans, celery leaves, spinach, and salami (if using), and stir.

Pour the whole mixture to a boil and stir for about 2 minutes.

Enjoy the soup hot!

Nutrition Info: Calories: 888, Total Fat: 19.9 g, Saturated Fat: 6.3 g, Cholesterol: 30 mg, Sodium: 1200 mg, Total Carbohydrate: 139.5 g, Dietary Fiber: 31.8 g, Total Sugars: 14.3 g, Protein: 49.4 g, Vitamin D: 14 mcg, Calcium: 64.3 mg, Iron: 22 mg, Potassium: 3951 mg

Baked Shrimp Stew

Servings: 4-6

Cooking Time: 25 Minutes

Ingredients:

Greek extra virgin olive oil

2 1/2 lb prawns, peeled, deveined, rinsed well and dried

1 large red onion, chopped (about two cups)

5 garlic cloves, roughly chopped

1 red bell pepper, seeded, chopped

2 15-oz cans diced tomatoes

1/2 cup water

1 1/2 tsp ground coriander

1 tsp sumac

1 tsp cumin

1 tsp red pepper flakes, more to taste

1/2 tsp ground green cardamom

Salt and pepper, to taste

1 cup parsley leaves, stems removed

1/3 cup toasted pine nuts

1/4 cup toasted sesame seeds

Lemon or lime wedges to serve

Directions:

Preheat the oven to 375 degrees F

In a large frying pan, add 1 tbsp olive oil

Sauté the prawns for 2 minutes, until they are barely pink, then remove and set aside

In the same pan over medium-high heat, drizzle a little more olive oil and sauté the chopped onions, garlic and red bell peppers for 5 minutes, stirring regularly

Add in the canned diced tomatoes and water, allow to simmer for 10 minutes, until the liquid reduces, stir occasionally

Reduce the heat to medium, add the shrimp back to the pan, stir in the spices the ground coriander, sumac, cumin, red pepper flakes, green cardamom, salt and pepper, then the toasted pine nuts, sesame seeds and parsley leaves, stir to combined

Transfer the shrimp and sauce to an oven-safe earthenware or stoneware dish, cover tightly with foil Place in the oven to bake for minutes, uncover and broil briefly.

allow the dish to cool completely

Distribute among the containers, store for 2-3 days

To Serve: Reheat on the stove for 1-2 minutes or until heated through. Serve with your favorite bread or whole grain. Garnish with a side of lime or lemon wedges.

Nutrition Info: Calories:377;Carbs: ;Total Fat: 20g;Protein: 41g

Mediterranean Pork Pita Sandwich

Servings: 6

Cooking Time: 10 Minutes

Ingredients:

2 teaspoons olive oil, plus 1 tablespoon

2 cups packed baby spinach leaves, finely chopped

4 ounces mushrooms, finely chopped

1 teaspoon chopped garlic

1 pound extra-lean ground pork

1 large egg

½ cup panko bread crumbs

⅓ cup chopped fresh dill

¼ teaspoon kosher salt

6 large romaine lettuce leaves, ripped into pieces to fit pita

2 tomatoes, sliced

3 whole-wheat pitas, cut in half

¾ cup Garlic Yogurt Sauce

Directions:

Heat 2 teaspoons of oil in a -inch skillet over medium heat. Once the oil is shimmering, add the spinach, mushrooms, and garlic and sauté for 3 minutes. Cool for 5 minutes.

Place the mushroom mixture in a large mixing bowl and add the pork, egg, bread crumbs, dill, and salt. Mix with your hands until everything is well combined. Make 6 patties, about ½-inch thick and 3 inches in diameter.

Heat the remaining 1 tablespoon of oil in the same 12-inch skillet over medium-high heat. When the oil is hot, add the patties. They should all be able to fit in the pan. If not, cook in 2 batches. Cook for 5 minutes on the first side and 4 minutes on the second side. The outside should be golden brown, and the inside should no longer be pink.

Place 1 patty in each of 6 containers. In each of 6 separate containers that will not be reheated, place 1 torn lettuce leaf and 2 tomato slices. Wrap the pita halves in plastic wrap and place one in each veggie container. Spoon 2 tablespoons of yogurt sauce into each of 6 sauce containers.

STORAGE: Store covered containers in the refrigerator for up to days. Uncooked patties can be frozen for up to 4 months, while cooked patties can be frozen for up to 3 months.

Nutrition Info: Total calories: 309; Total fat: 11g; Saturated fat: 3g; Sodium: 343mg; Carbohydrates: 22g; Fiber: 3g; Protein: 32g

SAUCES AND DRESSINGS RECIPES

Pomegranate Vinaigrette

Servings: ½ Cup

Cooking Time: 5 Minutes

Ingredients:

⅓ cup pomegranate juice

1 teaspoon Dijon mustard

1 tablespoon apple cider vinegar

½ teaspoon dried mint

2 tablespoons plus 2 teaspoons olive oil

Directions:

Place the pomegranate juice, mustard, vinegar, and mint in a small bowl and whisk to combine.

Whisk in the oil, pouring it into the bowl in a thin steam.

Pour the vinaigrette into a container and refrigerate.

STORAGE: Store the covered container in the refrigerator for up to 2 weeks. Bring the vinaigrette to room temperature and shake before serving.

Nutrition Info: Per Serving (2 tablespoons): Total calories: 94; Total fat: 10g; Saturated fat: 2g; Sodium: 30mg; Carbohydrates: 3g; Fiber: 0g; Protein: 0g

Green Olive And Spinach Tapenade

Servings: 1½ Cups

Cooking Time: 20 Minutes

Ingredients:

1 cup pimento-stuffed green olives, drained

3 packed cups baby spinach

1 teaspoon chopped garlic

½ teaspoon dried oregano

⅓ cup packed fresh basil

2 tablespoons olive oil

2 teaspoons red wine vinegar

Directions:

Place all the ingredients in the bowl of a food processor and pulse until the mixture looks finely chopped but not puréed. Scoop the tapenade into a container and refrigerate.
STORAGE: Store the covered container in the refrigerator for up to 5 days.

Nutrition Info: Per Serving (¼ cup): Total calories: 80; Total fat: 8g; Saturated fat: 1g; Sodium: 6mg; Carbohydrates: 1g; Fiber: 1g; Protein: 1g

GREAT MEDITERRANEAN DIET RECIPES

Grilled lemon chicken skewers

Preparation time: 10 minutes

Cooking time: 10 minutes

Servings: 6

Ingredients:

Two boneless chicken breasts

Seven green onions

Four minced garlic cloves

Three lemons

1 tbsp dried oregano

1 tsp kosher salt

1/4 cup olive oil

1/2 tsp black pepper

Directions :

Whisk salt, lemon juice, olive oil, garlic, lemon zest, black pepper, oregano, and sliced chicken pieces in a bowl.
Set aside for four hours.
Thread chicken, onions, and lemon slices onto the skewer.

Grill chicken skewers for 15 minutes on preheated grill over medium flames with often turning.
Serve when chicken is fully cooked.

Nutrition Info: Calories: 142 kcal Fat: 1 g Protein: 16 g Carbs: 3 g Fiber: 1 g

Black-eyed peas salad

Preparation time: 10-15 minutes
Cooking time: 15-20 minutes
Servings: 1

Ingredients:

One and a half cups black-eyed peas.
Half tsp of salt.
3/4 cup of chopped bell pepper.
Half tsp of freshly ground black pepper.
Half cup chopped celery.
1/4 cup of olive oil.
1 tbsp of sugar.
One clove of minced garlic.
2 tbsp of vinegar.

Directions :

Combine peas, celery, green bell pepper & onion in a bowl and mix.
Add oil, salt, sugar, vinegar, garlic, and black pepper in a bowl and mix with a fork.
Pour this dressing over vegetables.
Mix well.
Add hot sauce according to taste.

Toss to combine and put for a whole night.

The dish is ready to serve.

Nutrition Info: Calories: 324 kcal Fat: 11 g Protein: 5 g Carbs: 17 g Fiber: 4 g

Chicken shawarma pitas

Preparation time: 10 minutes
Cooking time: 30 minutes
Servings: 6

Ingredients:
¾ tbsp cumin
¾ tbsp coriander
¾ tbsp turmeric powder
One sliced onion
¾ tbsp garlic powder
½ tsp cloves
¾ tbsp paprika
1 tbsp lemon juice
½ tsp cayenne pepper
Eight boneless chicken
Salt to taste
1/3 cup olive oil
Pita bread
Tahini sauce

Directions :
In a bowl, add sliced chicken pieces, onions, cumin, garlic, cloves, olive oil, turmeric, paprika, lemon juice, salt, and

coriander. Toss well to coat chicken evenly. Set aside for three hours in the refrigerator.

Transfer the chicken pieces along with the marinade in a baking tray sprayed with oil.

Bake in a preheated oven at 425 degrees for 30 minutes.

Spread tahini sauce in pita bread and add baked chicken pieces. You can also add your favorite salad.

Serve and enjoy it.

Nutrition Info: Calories: 320 kcal Fat: 15.4 g Protein: 39.8 g Carbs: 4.3 g Fiber: 12 g

Sautéed chicken with olives capers and lemons

Preparation time: 5 minutes
Cooking time: 30 minutes
Servings: 4

Ingredients:
Six boneless chicken thighs
Two sliced lemons
One minced garlic clove minced
2/4 cup extra virgin olive oil
2 tbsp all-purpose flour
2 tbsp butter
1 cup chicken broth
kosher salt to taste
3/4 cup Sicilian green olives
2 tbsp parsley
1/4 cup capers
Black pepper to taste

Directions : Add salt, chicken, and pepper in a bowl and toss well. Set aside for 15 minutes.
Cook lemon slices (half of them) in heated olive oil over medium flame for five minutes from both sides.

Shift the cooked brown lemon slices on the plate.

Coat chicken pieces with rice flour and cook in heated olive oil in the skillet for seven minutes from both sides. Transfer the cooked chicken to the plate.

Sauté garlic in heated oil in the same pan for about half a minute. Stir in olives, chicken broth, lemons, and capers. Cook over high flame for few minutes.

When half of the broth is left, add parsley and butter. Cook for one minute.

Add salt and pepper to adjust the taste and serve.

Nutrition Info: Calories: 595 kcal Fat: 34 g Protein: 51 g Carbs: 5.5 g Fiber: 9 g

Spanish rice casserole with cheesy beef

Preparation time: 10 minutes
Cooking time: 25 minutes
Servings: 4

Ingredients:

16.8 oz Spanish Rice mix
1 tbsp olive oil
One red bell pepper
1 cup of corn
1 cup meatless crumbles
1/3 cup sour cream
1/4 cup salsa
1/2 cup Monterey Jack cheese
2 tbsp crumbled queso fresco
One avocado sliced

Directions :

Prepare the rice in a 2.5-liter casserole dish, which should be microwavable.

Preheat the microwave up to 375 F. Take a skillet and heat the oil. Now cook bell pepper till tendered 5-7 minutes. Once the rice is cooked, then combine the bell pepper, cooked, meatless crumbles, salsa, sour cream & corn. Now sprinkle the cheese on the top. Bake it, uncovered (10 minutes), till the cheese is melted & browned on top. Top sliced avocado.

Nutrition Info: Calories: 437 kcal Fat: 22 g Protein: 13 g Carbs: 46 g Fiber: 6 g

www.ingramcontent.com/pod-product-compliance
Lightning Source LLC
Chambersburg PA
CBHW070730030426
42336CB00013B/1930